HOSPITAL KNOW-HOW

A RESIDENCY GUIDE

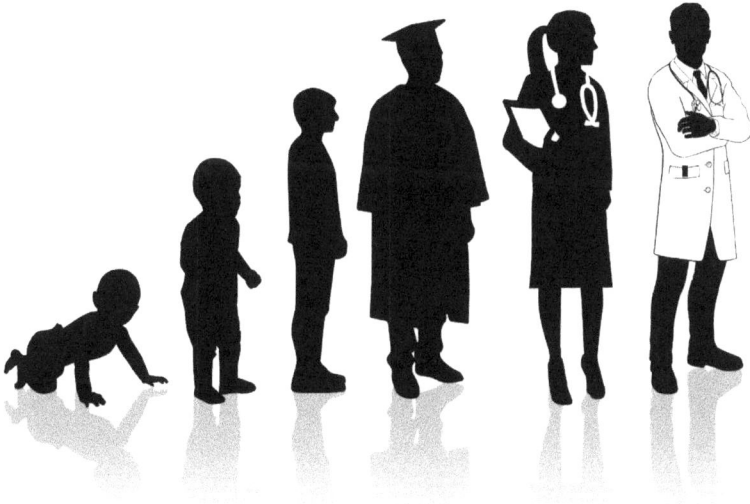

OMER ALSHEIKH M.D. | JAAFAR ELNAGAR M.D.

ISBN: 979-8-218-00817-8 (Paperback)
ISBN: 979-8-218-01128-4 (E-Book)

Cover and interior design Andy Meaden meadencreative.com

Contact the author at: Hospitalknowhow@gmail.com

First printing edition 2022.

Dedication

"In the name of Allah, the most gracious and the most merciful."
"My Lord, expand for me my breast [with assurance] and ease
for me my task and untie the knot from my tongue that they
may understand my speech."

—Surah Ta-Ha Ayat 25-28

I dedicate this guide to all future physicians, hoping it will ease
their evolution into becoming exceptional clinicians.

Contents

Preface

Congratulations on making it this far! Whether you're an incoming resident or medical student, this book speaks to all—both IMGs (international medical graduates) and AMGs (American medical graduates). I believe that if you have picked up this book and paused to question, *Will this be useful?* then you have already sensed its utility.

Who am I to believe that I know best about what you should know or be doing? I am neither a program director nor a faculty physician, but I have reason to believe that I understand your plight better than most, and can at the very least begin to guide you—learning from the great Greek philosopher Aristotle, who once said: "Well begun, is half done."

I believe that this kind of endeavor, a professional guide, should be undertaken by someone who can grasp your mindset. As an international medical graduate who had an enjoyable residency and successfully navigated its many trials and tribulations, I hope that my experiences may shed light on your journey to graduation.

I want to start by asking that you forgive my verbosity here in the Preface, but I wish to explain the origins of this book. I chose to write this book because of the profound lack of guidance I found before starting my residency. I am a medical student graduate from Sudan; I studied at the University of Medical Sciences and Technology (UMST) and had little idea of what I was getting myself into—all I knew was that I wanted to learn and practice the best medicine, which led me back to the United States.

Notice that I said "back". My story is slightly unorthodox: I did a lot of moving around growing up. I was born in Denver, Colorado, USA, moved to Oklahoma, New York, overseas to the United Arab Emirates, Sudan, and then to Detroit, Michigan, USA. Being exposed to and living within various cultures, I gained a communication, understanding, and adaptability skillset that became my lifeline during residency.

Studying medicine in Sudan was a handicap in my return to work in the USA, but it was also not without its benefits. I finished medical training straight from high school in a short five years, and the tuition cost was a mere fraction of studying in the USA. It was the obvious choice in terms of time and money, but the differences in practice and curriculum I would have to compensate for were daunting. A curriculum that is more focused on endemic tropical diseases like malaria is nowhere near the pathology I would need to know to work in the USA. Thus, I self-studied whilst juggling both curricula.

During my third year, I decided that I would take my USMLEs during university and apply for the residency match my graduating year. It was no simple task, but medicine is medicine at the end of the day. A few of my colleagues, namely Dr. Jaafar Elnagar and Dr. Ahmed Arrayeh, joined me on this journey, further spurring me on. We completed Step 1, Step 2 CS, and Step 2 CK during our fourth and fifth years. We graduated and came to the USA to begin our journey into residency.

We stumbled around at the start, attempting to figure out the application process. We soon started studying FREIDA & ERAS to see what was expected of us. We were horrified, realizing how underqualified we were to start residency. After working in outpatient clinics, we realized clinical practice here is incomparably different from Sudan, adding insult to injury. By the grace of God, we managed to secure interviews and match into our respective specialties.

Given that we had rotated through various specialties as part of our graduation requirement as sub-interns, we thought we would know how things should work. We didn't. This was evidenced by our ignorance during our clinical observerships. With little knowledge of what was to come, we began our frantic search to learn more about residency.

It began with online forums, hunting for advice, resources, and really any form of help. We looked for books and documents for guidance but couldn't find anything of substance. We first sought out medical knowledge, so we re-read our medical school references and took the STEP 3 exam, hoping it would give us some insight. Despite this refreshment of our medical knowledge, we were still ill-prepared for intern year.

We suffered from a significant deficiency: hospital know-how.

We were full of zeal but severely lacking in knowledge. Hospital know-how is the first deficiency of an intern, and as we came to learn—*the dedicated do improve.* The second deficiency is medical knowledge. Regarding these shortcomings, I imperatively stress the following point: *there is no shame in saying that you do not know.* The practice of medicine is a world apart from the study of medicine.

My personal experience was exceptional; I started at absolute zero. Information overload quickly set in, as did imposter syndrome. I started on one of the most challenging rotations of my residency, night float at Ascension St. John's hospital. I had to learn how to do everything quickly and correctly. I was blessed to have some of the strongest senior residents as my first seniors. They were patient, helpful, and knowledgeable. Seeing how efficient and accurate they were made me think, am I the right person for the job? Was I going to be functioning at that level in two short years? I could not believe it.

Sitting here now, I know it is doable—despite how daunting it may seem. The concerted effort of all my seniors and attendings gave me the skills I needed to excel. I progressed well and was soon on level ground with the other residents who had rotated in the USA prior. Intern year was not without its struggles. As a good friend of mine would say, "The hard is what makes it great."

At the end of my intern year, I was awarded "Intern of the Year", although I believe I would've been a better fit for a Most Improved Resident award. As I progressed, I tried to teach all that I knew to new interns and medical students alike. Upon graduation, I received the "Resident of the Year" award. I am currently working at Massachusetts General Brigham, Salem, hospital as a hospitalist and aspire to pursue a cardiology fellowship.

As an intern, you must remember seniors and attendings want you to learn. A strong intern is one of the prized possessions of a residency program as they almost always continue to excel in their career. They propel patient care, the teams they work on, and the name of their program to new heights. As doctors, we are destined to teach. That innate drive, to elevate the following generation of physicians, led me to write this book.

I have structured this book in a chronological ascent into the responsibilities of residency. Thus, it starts in the sense of learning to be an intern, progressing from proverbial clinical infancy: crawling and cooing, to walking and talking.

I hope you understand my and this book's deficiencies, as I can only explain how I see fit, and use my success as the standard of proof. Furthermore, the descriptions, terms, and explanations I give are all colored by my own experiences and my residency's structure. The definitions and usage will vary by hospital and specialty. I have made an earnest attempt to make this as general a guide as possible—to avoid making this book specifically about internal medicine intern year.

For this reason, I must give credit where it is due. The contributions of Dr. Jaafar Elnagar, an aspiring colorectal surgeon; Dr. Mustafa Ali, a soon-to-be Pulmonology/Critical Care fellow; and Dr. Mahasin Tariq, a soon-to-be Neonatology fellow, have helped me stay true to the goal of this book.

As I discussed with my friends, if we succeed in lightening the load and lighting the path for you throughout your intern year, then we have reached our intended goal.

Acknowledgements

First and foremost, I would like to say all praise and thanks to Allah (SWT).

To my mother: Hala Elhoweris, and my father: Negmeldin Alsheikh, words fail to describe my gratitude, so I will strive to show it to you in my actions for the rest of my life.

To my younger brothers, you guys are pretty much useless, but I know I'll get an earful for not being inclusive, so small thanks.

I am grateful for my extended family, friends, and mentors. The guidance and patience you all exerted to curtail my flight of ideas into a structured, sensible human production are appreciated.

A special thanks to my colleagues Dr. Mahasin Tariq and Dr. Mustafa Ali for their influential role in critiquing and reviewing this book to ensure it was inclusive and relevant.

Last but not least, I thank you, the reader. Without you in mind, this book would never have come to fruition. I commend your zeal and dedication to excellence.

PART ONE
TO TALK

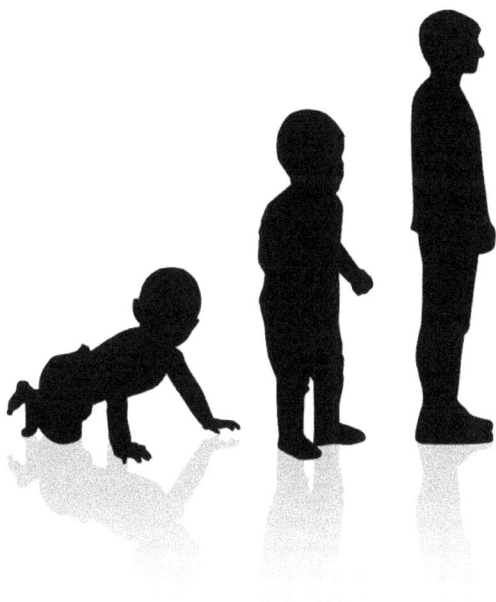

Chapter 1

Medical Mentality and Learning to Talk

Before starting residency, you should first understand the mentality with which it should be approached. Remember, this is not the end of your medical education journey; it is the beginning of it.

Medical school does its part by supplying you with the medical knowledge needed to practice to the best of its ability. How much you retain and can apply is within your power, but as I said in the Preface, medical knowledge is the second deficiency; hospital know-how is the first.

The medical mindset to excel

The first order of business is grasping that you are, in fact, deficient, and embracing this with humility. We all start out ignorant. Nobody graduates from medical school as an attending or a specialist. Even if you did practice abroad at an advanced level, you are still unaware of your hospital's particular system. Yes, you are ignorant, as am I. We are all ignorant but in different aspects and at different levels. You must start with the initial belief that your seniors and attendings know better. That being said, different viewpoints on a case should be voiced and we will discuss how to do this correctly later.

The second order of business is understanding your role. You do not start out dictating patient management plans and calling the shots. You build your way up to that. In the beginning, you learn the very basics of patient care. "Scut work," as it is unlovingly called, is beneficial.

Learning to do basic things, be it "getting numbers," blood draws, writing notes, presenting patients, talking to other team members, and having family discussions, are all essential parts of the process. Learning to do these well is a crucial step in your progression to seniority. Seeing each patient and task as a burden only undermines your residency experience. On the other hand, viewing each opportunity as a learning experience allows you to learn rapidly while extracting all the benefits of residency.

The third order of business is performing your duties with diligence. You are in training, and it is understandable to feel overwhelmed by your ignorance. As an intern, you will be challenged; this is a necessary part of your development. As always remember, "the dedicated do improve" and repetition will make you more efficient in your day-to-day tasks if you do them with presence.

Therefore, laziness is the enemy. Do your best to avoid complacency in your duties. Seniors and attendings effortlessly recognize those who want to learn compared to those trying to "fly under the radar." Nobody will fault you for not knowing initially, especially if it's your first attempt at a case or procedure. Although, if you are struggling in a particular area, it should be your primary concern to correct it.

What you want out of residency is quite evident in your work ethic. Those who wish to succeed show it. It is also a matter of teachability. Those who want to learn are taught easily compared to those who don't. Being lazy or, even worse, being *labeled* lazy is never a good thing. You could suffer from that impression for the length of your residency and receive worse treatment and teaching from others based on that alone. It is not right, but it is in our faulty human nature to reciprocate effort at times.

The fourth order of business is correcting the possible misconceptions and misgivings you may already harbor towards residency. It is a difficult phase of training, without a doubt, but it takes work to make a physician out of a raw mass of medical knowledge. Remember, the whole point of residency is for you to learn, and although as you progress, you may become "jaded," you are still, in essence, a student. Leave your ego at the door and try your best to improve. Once you graduate, finding someone to learn from becomes more and more difficult.

The laws of practice

This discussion leads us into what I call the *Laws of Practice*. These apply not only to you but to any physician, at any level, anywhere.

You Must:

1. **Never lie**—to patients nor team members. Be responsible for things you have done or mistakes you have made. Only by acknowledging them first can you grow from them. Always communicate with a higher-up if you believe you've done something wrong. Lying in any shape or form will get you in trouble. *The worst form is within patient care. Lying within this realm can result in poor outcomes for patients.* Therefore, it is the most serious offense you can commit. For example, lying about the patient's history.

2. **Prioritize patient care**—always prioritize the patients' best interests. Their well-being is why we do what we do. Also, respect their wishes (if they are competent) even if they contradict best medical practice and *always try to understand the why to their decisions.*

3. **Communicate respectfully**—to all team members, caregivers, and anybody you meet on your journey. We are all part of a system that works to take care of people, and flawed as it may be, it's working. Try to explain why you are doing something to co-patients and other staff if time allows.

4. **Never judge**—patients/ co-patients in any shape, way, or form in which they may differ from yourself or the society you identify with. You may understand medical problems but are probably ignorant of the intricate issues affecting a patient at a specific point in their life.

5. **Improve**—this is a duty to all our patients, to advance our medical practices for their betterment. Any shape, way, or form of improvement is a step forward, even if it is a personal one.

Guiding principles and goals

Throughout residency, you will hear that the goal is to make you a safe doctor. I agree with this as a goal, but believe it is a meager goal. Granted, depending on your specialty this can mean wildly different things—for a surgeon to be safe is different from an internist, and so on. The way I see it, your goal should be more robust. You should aim to be an accurate, efficient, *and* safe doctor.

Of course, the primordial fear of a physician should be to wrong a patient. To misdiagnose, mistreat and mislabel a patient *out of negligence* can be seen as a fundamental failure as a physician. The classification of errors into commission and omission is imperative to our field.

We should never commit errors with intent and should never commit errors out of negligence. Alas, "To err is human" and errors are inevitable. Nevertheless, the difference lies here: a mistake that occurs out of ignorance is forgivable if the correct steps were taken to avoid it.

Thus, the first guideline—*If you don't know, ask.*

This leads us to the second guideline. Medicine is hierarchical. We have a chain of command, and work may be divided according to rank. The orders that come down should be followed. That being said, we are encouraged to have open discussions, and mutual respect is vital for good practice.

Thus, the second guideline—*Do as you are told.*

As an intern, you will most likely have medical students under you. Your duty to them is to teach what you know and lend them a helping hand on their journey as well. As you progress into seniority, the list of those under you will expand over your career. To improve care, we must improve as physicians, and to that end, we must teach.

Thus, the third guideline—*What you know, teach.*

My goal is to make you an excellent intern, right? As such, I asked you to set a loftier goal; but what is an accurate, effective, and safe clinician? Those three words, to me, mean the world in terms of patient care. Efficiency and accuracy as a physician have their own nuance. It means not only are you capable of seeing patients, formulating care plans, and enacting them, but you can do so quickly and correctly. To be safe is the art of avoiding mistakes of commission, omission, and correctable ignorance.

Efficiency foremost is to act and carry out tasks with the best use of time possible. This applies to everything you do. Be it taking a history, writing notes, presenting patients, etc. The American medical system moves at a rapid pace. You will probably learn to speed-walk in your first year, as many of us now do without thinking.

Of course, there are ways to be fast and still be cordial. You should never rush a patient or nurse who is voicing their concerns. It is up to you to control the pace of your work and optimize where you can. You will get faster, and that takes time. Make sure that a conscious goal of yours is to care for patients more efficiently— without sacrificing quality.

Accuracy is the ability to secure the correct diagnosis and act on it. Note that efficiency comes *before* accuracy, as getting the proper diagnosis too late is, in essence, useless to the patient. You should always use all your faculties when evaluating a patient. The history, physical examination, lab work, and imaging studies are your prized tools. The first way to improve as a clinician is by using these tools well.

These are the tools that will allow your medical knowledge to guide you to the correct diagnosis, after which you can begin to treat and care for a patient. Getting it right to the best of your ability should be your goal. Although you should not stray from the guidelines and laws mentioned earlier in your efforts, as we note, there are very complex and complicated cases in the medical field. We do not always have the correct answers, and that is fine. If you have exerted your tools appropriately, that is all anyone can ask of you.

The vocabulary of practice

To use these tools and reach our diagnosis and treatment goals, you must be able to navigate the language of hospital communication. Let's move forward into learning the vocabulary of practice.

The following is a list I've compiled consisting of terms, definitions, and acronyms commonly used across hospitals in different regions of the country. Overall, the usage will be the same, and committing the following list to memory will serve you well.

The general terms are broadly grouped by the following attributes A. Hospital logistics, B. People, and C. Places. The common acronyms on the other hand follow a logical progression or grouping based on their utility or specialty

General terms

A. Hospital Logistics—*Everyday terms encountered that pertain to patient care and hospital management.*

Admission—The act of accepting a patient to be treated in the hospital.

Inpatient—A level of care, meaning the patient will be admitted for more than two mid-nights most of the time. It may also be a general term for a patient admitted to the hospital.

Observation—A level of care, meaning the patient will be admitted for one midnight for monitoring. Based on how a patient is doing and the severity of illness, the level of care may be changed.

Transfer—The act of moving a patient from one place to another. It can be between hospitals or from one part of the hospital to another. Example: ICU transfer. Has many other similar terms (Downgrade: out of ICU; Upgrade: to the ICU).

Discharge—DC, the act of releasing a patient safely as medically planned from the hospital to the outside world. Patients may be discharged to many different places, which are noted below.

Service—Team of providers, usually classified by specialty. Example: Trauma service, medicine service, etc. The admitting or primary service is the first team taking and caring for the patient during their admission.

Electronic health record—EHR or electronic medical record, EMR, where a patient's information is stored and interacted with. It is through this application we facilitate the treatment and care of patients. For a specific patient, it is known as their chart.

Medical record number—MRN, a patient identification number.

Date of birth—DOB, patient's birth date.

Orders—1. The act of placing an electronic "message" to other care team members that something must be done. It may be written, typed or verbalized through a nurse. Example: order an echo, order a diet, order insulin, order a thoracentesis. 2. An area in the chart that shows what was done, what is currently active, and what will be done for a patient's treatment plan (medications, imaging, lab work, procedures, etc.)

Bolus—A single dose of a drug or other medicinal preparation given all at once, for example, 1 liter lactated ringers fluid bolus. It can also be a small rounded portion of an object, like a food bolus.

Lab work—The patient's test results can be from any bodily fluid or sample. They are usually revised chronologically from the current date and compared to prior results. Also called "numbers."

Imaging/radiology—Imaging studies such as X-rays, CTs, and MRIs. Specific EMR/EHR charts have subsets for cardiovascular studies or procedures, e.g., echoes, colonoscopies, etc.

History and physical—H&P, the initial encounter and documentation with a patient by the *admitting service*. A complete history and physical examination, with a documented management plan.

Discharge summary—DC summary is documentation of the hospital stay by the inpatient team (usually by the admitting service), reviewed by attendings with or without senior residents. It is read by a physician in the outpatient setting to understand the patient's hospital stay and facilitate the transition of care.

Chief complaint—C.C, the patient's primary complaint that brings them to the hospital.

History of presenting illness—HPI, the patient's history, in their own words, relevant to their current or recent admissions.

Review of systems—ROS, history of other bodily systems.

Physical examination—An organ system-based examination of patients and their signs.

Assessment and plan—A&P or A/P, the list of diagnoses and treatment plans. This includes different structures and varies by residency/specialty/role. Also known as impression and plan.

Follow up—Seeing a patient again or checking on something again. This term may be used in both outpatient and inpatient settings.

Notes—Varied types of clinical documentation, briefly divided into progress notes (PN), consultation (CN), H&P, E.D provider or visit, significant event, nursing notes, etc.

SOAP note—Subjective, objective, assessment, and plan note.

Progress note—PN, documentation of a focused assessment on how the patient is doing today compared to yesterday; done for follow up, usually in SOAP format.

Consultation note—CN, documentation of a focused but full history and exam, relevant to consulting service on questions or concerns from the primary service.

Sign-out—To report in a summarized fashion to a covering resident. Usually verbal with the use of a hand-off.

Hand-off—A paper or electronic document on which the sign-out is written to summarize the patient and their hospital stay.

Cross-coverage—To cover (take care of) different teams from your own. Usually within the same specialty.

Code Status—The course of action to be taken when someone is in cardiorespiratory arrest, usually either FULL CODE—you may intubate and resuscitate the patient with chest compressions; or DNR/DNI—do not perform intubation or compressions, also known as "heroic measures" and allow the patient to pass.

Code Blue—The cardiorespiratory arrest of an adult, a medical alert. Different hospitals have various coding systems for pediatric arrests and obstetric emergencies. Blue is the most consistent code nationwide. Study your hospital's system before starting.

Section 12—A document filled out by a physician regarding a patient that needs to be involuntarily committed for no more than 72 hours. For example, suicidal patients.

B. People—*The people and teams who are involved in the clinical care and discharge planning of patients.*

Co-patient—Family or friend accompanying patient who may be physically present or contacted via phone.

Health care proxy—HCP, medical decision-maker for a patient. If a patient is deemed incompetent or does not have capacity, decision-making for the patient goes to them. It can be set in the outpatient setting or discussed when the patient is competent. Usually, the point of contact for updates.

Attending physician—The supervising physician primarily in charge of the patient's case. The clinical hierarchal rank abroad comparatively is the consultant as they are specialists in their field.

Consultant physician—A consulting physician is usually from a specialized service. Example: cardiologist, vascular surgeon, neurosurgeon. They may be primary in some instances, in which case the physician in charge is the attending.

Resident—Physician in training usually refers to a person in their second year, and onward.

Intern—A first-year resident. They may not always be called residents. They are sometimes referred to as interns or PGY-1 (postgraduate year 1) alone.

Senior resident—A resident beyond their first year of training. When you are called a senior varies based on hospital and residency.

Chief resident—Can be a newly graduated full-fledged attending with supervisory responsibilities for the residency program. They may also be an exceptional senior resident with those same extra responsibilities. In general surgery, all residents who reach their fifth year are chiefs. Their roles and stages vary from program to program. They are excellent resources of information and help.

Staff or faculty—Physicians involved in teaching residents and managing a residency program.

Program Director—P.D, The physician in overall charge of a residency program.

Associate Program Director—A physician in charge of certain parts of the residency program who assists the P.D in their responsibilities.

Program Coordinator—A person whose role is to keep the residency functioning smoothly; they have many talents and functions. Usually, an excellent resource for things you need or trouble you may have at the start. Can connect you with the appropriate people.

Chief Medical Officer—A physician who works from the administrative side of the hospital to improve patient care and hospital standards etc.

Chief of Medicine/Surgery/Pediatrics/Ob-gyn—Heads of their departments, respectively.

Hospitalist—A physician who specializes in caring for admitted patients only. They may be an Internal Medicine (I.M), Pediatrics (Peds), or Family Medicine (F.M) physician in their specialization.

Primary Care Physician—PCP, a physician who specializes in the care of patients in the primary care setting, such as clinics, and oversees most of the patient's care. Usually, I.M, F.M, or Peds physicians.

Physician Assistant—P.A, a person who has studied a Master's degree to practice clinically under supervision from a physician. They have learned medical concepts and may also function like interns/residents, such as seeing patients, writing notes, etc.

Social Worker—SW, a person who functions as a liaison between patients, their families, and hospital discharge resources. Example: primary care clinics, drug rehabilitation centers, etc.

Case Manager—CM, works closely with the social worker and may help with the discharge placement of a patient into rehabilitation centers. They can also provide patients with resources on discharge, such as wheelchairs, walkers, oxygen, and the like.

Nurses—RN or registered nurse. Function: to care for patients; they administer medications and monitor patients. Act as our eyes and ears.

SWAT RN—Nurses specialized in caring for critical patients, like ICU nurses, very skilled the majority of the time.

Nurse Practitioner—NP, a nurse with further training in a specific specialty, does not care for patients in the traditional nurse sense but works under a specialist attending similar responsibilities to an intern/resident or PA. Gaining more independence in clinical practice. Varies by state. Also known as mid-level or advanced care practitioner.

Patient Care Technician—PCT, helps RNs care for patients, usually obtaining vital signs, blood sugars, and assisting in moving patients.

Physical Therapy—PT, a specialty whereby physical therapists train patients on major bodily movements. Think big joints or gross movements. For example, gait, standing up, sitting down, etc. They help decide where patients are discharged to.

Occupational Therapy—OT, a specialty whereby occupational therapists train patients on "Micro movements," think smaller joints. For example, opening pill bottles, picking things up, etc. Usually, work with physical therapy in deciding discharge planning for patients.

Speech Therapy—A specialty whereby speech therapists train patients on swallowing safety and speaking techniques. For example, stroke patients or elderly demented patients. They assist in diet consistency choices during hospital admissions.

Respiratory Therapy—A specialty whereby respiratory therapists place patients on ventilatory assist devices (CPAP, BIPAP), assist with chest physiotherapy and pulmonary toileting via suctioning. May administer nebulized treatments and obtain arterial blood gases. Help optimize respiratory status during admission.

Phlebotomist—A person who specializes in drawing blood for tests. Nurses and residents do not typically draw blood, but this may vary depending on the hospital and scenario, such as ICU nurses, doctor-to-draw cases, etc.

Intravenous team—IV teams, usually RNs, specialized in placing difficult IV catheters or specialized catheters such as peripherally inserted central catheters (PICCs) or midline catheters.

Interventional radiologists—IR, physicians specialized in radiological techniques to perform procedures. Variable skill-set, do a high volume of cases daily, including biopsies, angiographies, thoracentesis (thoras), paracentesis (paras), etc. May not be present in all hospitals.

Critical Response Team—CRT, also known as RRT or rapid response team. A team comprises a physician, swat nurse, and patient's nurse responding to a decompensating or critical patient.

Emergency Medical Services—EMS, ambulances mostly. Anyone may bring patients in, including family, friends, the fire department, and the police.

Hospice—A service that provides care for patients at home, at a facility, or in the hospital. Focused on quality of life over quantity of life. Life expectancy is expected to be less than six months.

Palliative Care—End-of-life care, a medical specialty in and of itself. Multifaceted capabilities to assist with quality of life like hospice, inpatient teams assist in end-of-life discussions, pain management, etc.

Jane/John Doe—A patient with an unknown name and age, no known identifiers.

C. Places—*Various setting of patient care,*
both inpatient and outpatient

Operating room—O.R, the surgical suites where surgeries take place.

Intensive care unit—ICU, can be divided by specialty at times: CICU or CVICU—cardiac or cardiovascular ICU; SICU—surgical ICU; PICU—pediatric ICU; NICU—neonatal ICU.

Step Down Unit—SDU, ICU step down, or HDU as its known abroad. The SDU provides an intermediate level of care between ICU and the general medical floors. Provides higher trained nursing, and better nurse to patient ratios. The patient is severely ill if they are here but does not require ICU-level care.

Floors—The medical floors, medicine/surgical/pediatric/obstetrics, and gynecology (Ob-gyn) beds are here. Like the term "wards" abroad.

Emergency Department—E.D, also known as the Emergency Room—E.R.

EMS—Emergency Medical Services, ambulances mostly. Anyone may bring patients in, including family, friends, the fire department, and the police.

Triage—A place where patients are evaluated based on their severity of illness and assigned to respective units in the E.D.

Resuscitation or Trauma Bay—A place where the most critical patients are brought in on arrival to the E.D.

Labor and delivery—L&D, Ob-gyn ward

Ambulatory—Means a primary care setting, also known as outpatient, may also be a part of the E.D. with very low acuity (measurement of intensity of nursing care and patient triage).

Telemetry—Cardiac monitoring for heart rate and rhythm 24/7 while in the hospital. May refer to a cardiac floor.

Sub-Acute Rehabilitation—SAR, a facility where nursing staff, physical therapy, and basic medical care are offered. It can be attached to the hospital or at a SNF—skilled nursing facility. Patients may present from or be sent to these facilities. Sometimes called "nursing homes," however the use of that term has bad connotations for many people.

Inpatient Rehabilitation—IPR, usually a stand-alone facility where more intense physical therapy is available, may also be in the hospital. Usually needs a PMR (physical medicine and rehabilitation) doctor's evaluation in addition to PT/OT. (SAR and IPR may be interchangeable terms based on geography). The majority of patients need neuromuscular training, for example, stroke or trauma patients.

Long-Term Acute Care—LTAC, a high level of care in which patients require significant support: ventilators, vasopressors, etc. Think of an ICU with a long-term stay.

Common Acronyms

Pt.—Patient

PMH—Past medical history

PSH—Past surgical history

SH or SHX—Social history

DH—Drug history

FH—Family history

DC—Discharge

RTL—Running the list, revising the patients and their care briefly

PRN—As needed

AMA—Against medical advice

BIBA—Brought in by ambulance

RL—Residents' lounge

PL—Physicians' lounge

MS—Medical student

OTC—Over the counter

Q*—How often something is done, e.g., Q8hrs=every 8 hours.

Ppx—Prophylaxis

Rx—Prescription

O_2—Oxygen

2/2—Secondary to

NC—Nasal cannula

NRB—Non-rebreather

Vent—Ventilator

ECMO—Extracorporeal membrane oxygenation

MAR—Medication administration record

DVT—Deep vein thrombosis

SCD—Sequential compression device

Dispo—Disposition, discharge planning for Pt.

CLABSI—Central line-associated bloodstream infection

CAUTI—Catheter-associated urinary tract infection

PE—Pulmonary embolism

CTAB—Clear to auscultation bilaterally

NAEON—No acute events overnight

SOCRATES—Site, onset, character, radiation, timing, exacerbating and relieving factors, severity. Hx-taking tool.

VSS—Vital signs stable

AXO—Alert and oriented, may be out of 3 or 4, e.g., AXO-3

R/O—Rule out

ROS—Review of systems

LOS—Length of stay

POD—Postoperative day

ISS—Insulin sliding scale

POC—Point of care (pinprick blood draw)

BS—Blood sugar

H&H—Hemoglobin and hematocrit

CBC—Complete blood count

BMP—Basic metabolic panel (electrolytes, BUN, and cr., RFTs)

CMP—Complete metabolic panel (Expanded BMP including albumin, LFTs, and bilirubin)

ABG—Arterial blood gas

VBG—Venous blood gas

CPAP—Continuous positive airway pressure

BIPAP—Bilevel positive airway pressure

Neb—Nebulized treatment

B/L—Bilaterally

BKA—Below knee amputation

AKA—Above-knee amputation

Ex Lap—Exploratory laparotomy

Appy—Appendectomy

Lap chole—Laparoscopic cholecystectomy

GSW—Gunshot wound

PROM—Premature rupture of the membranes

IVF—Intravenous fluids or in vitro fertilization

NWB—Non-weight bearing

PWB—Partial weight bearing

WBAT—Weight-bearing as tolerated

NPO—Nil per OS, nothing by mouth

PO—Oral

Feeding tube—via NG, PEG, or PEJ tubes

NGT—Nasogastric tube

NJT—Nasojejunal tube

PEG—Percutaneous endoscopic gastrostomy tube

PEJ—Percutaneous endoscopic jejunostomy tube

S/P—Status post

FTT—Failure to thrive

CP—Cerebral palsy

U/S—Ultrasound (May be US)

MRI—Magnetic resonance imaging

CT—Computed tomography

GDD/DD—Global developmental delay, developmental delay

B&D—Behavior and development

GA—Gestational age

STAT—Immediately

FYI— For your information

DNR—Do not resuscitate

DNI—Do not intubate

This serves as an elementary list for navigating documentation and care-team interactions. There is still a bank of terms that you'll primarily learn in the hospital that are specialty-specific. You should focus during rounds and when reading notes to pick them up. Drug trade names and acronyms for diseases or procedures are part of that paradigm.

A quick internet search will serve you well and, as always, use your friends and seniors in residency. At the very least, I believe this serves as a starting point with which you can at least begin to move towards *thinking* like a resident.

Chapter 2

Understanding Your Environment

Since you now understand some general terms, let us delve into specifics. Once you have matched, you will be bombarded with paperwork. After you navigate that battlefield, you may have some big decisions to make pertaining to your schedule for the following year. Not all residencies allow you to choose your schedule, but having a basic understanding of the rotations you will be starting on will help you immensely. Below are a few preliminary terms and definitions that will assist you in this regard.

Schedules, core rotations, and electives

ACGME: (Accreditation Council for Graduate Medical Education): The governing body of accreditation for all residencies in the United States. They make the rules that accredited programs must follow.

Core rotation: These are clinical rotations that are graduation requirements decided by the ACGME for your type of residency training. They are the foundation and bulk of residency training. In general, they're more work-intensive than elective rotations.

Call: Being on-call is the act of admitting and caring for patients in the hospital while covering other teams or residents. It can be just named call or split into long and short calls. Long call is usually a 24-hour shift; while short call may be an extra 2-4 hours after a standard day end (5 p.m.), the hours will vary based on specialty and hospital.

Back-up: A scheduling system for residents to be called in if another resident cannot perform their duties. It may be called jeopardy as well. The back-up resident must be available to get to the hospital quickly if called in.

Elective rotation: These are clinical rotations that you can choose from to enhance your training. However, some elective rotations are requirements for graduation; this can be dictated by ACGME or your residency program.

Vacation: Time off from all clinical duties.

X+Y: A system in which you work inpatient for X number of weeks and then in the outpatient clinics for Y number of weeks.

Nights/Night float: Nocturnal shifts consistently, usually for a few weeks to a month. It can also be one night when your team is on-call.

Onboarding: The act of completing paperwork, online modules, etc., before your residency start date.

Your first hurdle will be to obtain your licensing for onboarding; this should be done STAT. This helps the program get you settled in, as you need your training licenses and permissions before your start. Visa paperwork should also be done promptly. As you may already know, immigration is complicated and takes time. Earlier is better.

Each program will have specific names for its rotations, and I would be lying if I said I could recount them all. In general, you will have the majority of core rotations during intern year and possibly a few elective rotations. Rotations may be in 2-week blocks but are usually monthly.

As an example, for internal medicine rotations, the most common will be "floors" or "staff," which is your inpatient medicine rotation. They may also name rotations by parts of the hospital or specialty. In surgery, the equivalent may be called "chief rotation". The best way to understand your schedule is to ask a senior, a chief resident, or the program coordinator.

When it comes to starting on a new rotation, come early. You should always arrive early and start seeing your patients to prepare for rounds. You are expected to have seen your patients before the start of rounds. For example—rounds in ICU begin at 7 a.m., so you should come in at 6 a.m. to give yourself enough time to see your patients and familiarize yourself with their problems, treatment, and how they are doing today. An intern who comes late and is not prepared for rounds may have that reflected in their evaluations (Evals). We will discuss evals at the end of this book.

Vacations and emergencies

A quick note on vacations. These may be chosen or assigned to you. They are usually selected during elective rotations for most residencies. Depending on your program, national holidays can be half days, regular workdays, or off; this also varies based on your rotation. Vacations can be limited to 1-week blocks spread out over the year. Some residencies allow for larger blocks of time off, such as 2-4 weeks off as a block. Most residencies do not allow for more than four weeks off in an academic year.

Paternal and maternal leave varies from residency to residency. Discuss with your Program Coordinator if you or your family are expecting. Furthermore, we are all human, and emergencies do arise. Always communicate with your supervisors promptly should something happen to you or your family and you need *emergent* time off.

Do not use this lightly; it is intended for real emergencies. More often than not, if you are pulled off a core rotation, another resident will cover your position, with them likely being pulled from an elective rotation. You may need to make up the time lost for graduation requirements or "pay it back" towards that resident later.

Understanding your role

Now that you have an idea of where and how you will start, let's discuss your role. The roles of an intern are varied—of course, since you are at the beginning of your training and need to be exposed to all aspects of patient care to gain experience. Most intern responsibilities will include patient evaluations, note writing, placing orders, covering the team's pager or phone, learning procedures, attending conferences, and communicating with support staff, families, and patients.

Quite the long list, right? Don't worry—you will be capable of doing all this at some point. We still have a way to go and will delve into each of those responsibilities as we progress through this book.

Remember, your senior will be your lifeline when you start. They will be your prime resource and example. Learn the best you can from them. They will show you the way to the best of their ability. It is their duty, as we said earlier. Do not be afraid to ask questions but try to find answers yourself before asking—*if it is feasible.* For example: you can google what apixaban is, but do not be hesitant in asking your senior what to do with a hemorrhaging patient who takes it.

Questions that can be answered with a quick google search or the usage of medical information apps are best saved for those purposes. Other questions or concerns should be directed to your senior resident.

As you have understood the mentality, laws, and environment in which we practice, we can now say you *think* like a resident. Let us discuss the first part of learning: to *talk* like a resident.

Chapter 3

First Words, Gathering Information

The very first thing we should revise here is history taking. As we all know, a good history is the foundation of an accurate diagnosis. How is a history here different from abroad, you may ask? Efficiency, structure, and presentation are the primary differences. A complete history is mostly taken once during the admission process, but is also pertinent for transfers of care. Your account of the patient will be read and relied upon by every caregiver on the team. Do not take it lightly.

Revision of history taking and explanation of the SOAP format

Firstly, a good history is accurate to *the patient's account* of their disease process, and this must be consistent, chronological, and logical to the best of your ability. Not all patients are excellent historians, and not all diseases present themselves clearly. Thus, it is essential to build a systematic framework of history taking while extracting *a relevant history that concentrates* on *the condition we are treating now.*

I will not go into the details of history taking as I assume you know this already. I will leave you with these reminders: Always revise the history and see if it makes sense. If the patient cannot provide a narrative, *always do your best to find someone who can and take a complete account from them. Deficiencies in history result in deficiencies in care.* Also, document why they could not narrate their own history and list who provided it.

Secondly, a good history is efficient. Obtaining the correct information quickly and without making the patient feel rushed is the true art of history taking. Using the techniques mentioned below will help you in time management.

For example, if someone is admitted with abdominal pain, it is essential to note they had a lap-chole five days ago. You don't need to discuss in detail their chronic hypertension during this admission. Also, prioritize diseases and treatment plans in terms of severity. Superseding the patient's concerns might be necessary at times as they may not grasp the seriousness of their illnesses.

The structure of a history and its presentation may vary depending on the service you are on. Also, the specificity and depth of a particular disease process will change if you are a consulting team or the primary team. You will notice these differences soon into training. Most of the time, the structure should be consistent with the following eight points:

History structure:

1 C.C

2. *HPI- Starting with the patient's age, race, and RELEVANT PMH. The C.C with the associated symptoms and story. Application of SOCRATES, ROS, etc.*

3. *Past medical history—rest of diseases.*

4. *Past surgical history—recent is more valuable than remote.*

5. *Family history—relevant to the disease being worked up or treated.*

6. *Drug history—current medications are vital and must be known. Recently stopped medications should also be mentioned.*

7. *Allergies—medication and type of allergy. (Many patients list side effects as allergies.)*

8. *Social history—social habits must be known in detail.*

As a matter of preference, I disagree with removing race in the HPI like some physicians do. As we know, some diseases are associated with specific races. I also can't entirely agree with using the descriptive terms "pleasant" and "gentleman/woman", as although the patient may be this, the lack of usage in other notes may lead people to believe that other patients are unpleasant, etc.

When taking the history, allow the patient to tell their story, but you must be an effective history taker. We all start off slow, taking more time with patients than we may have to offer. Time management is something to be worked on as you progress. Do not rush through the history without being tactful. A patient will know if you are being impatient with them.

Your tools are many, such as redirecting the patient to the main history and using silence to prompt them to refocus if they continue to be tangential. Always actively listen as they will feel more comfortable providing information to you. Never give them the sense that you judge them for their actions, even if they are detrimental to their health. Guide them to making the right decisions at the right time. Use your sense of when to discuss specific things, and always be honest and reassuring. We are here for them at the end of the day.

Let us move on to the SOAP format. It is the backbone of a progress note, which documents a follow-up visit. The utility of the progress note lies in the documentation of the patient's case on a day-by-day basis. The progress note will demonstrate the plan and show other team members how the patient feels and what is being done.

There are also fundamental points to be addressed by the primary team seeing the patient; they are summarized by one of my favorite attendings as peeing, pooing, and walking. Are they able to perform bodily functions on their own or not? These points will change management and discharge planning. It needs to be acted upon early during the admission. To be asked during the subjective and addressed in the A&P.

- **S**—*Subjective. How the patient feels. You should ask the patient questions relevant to their hospital stay. For someone admitted for a STEMI, you will ask about chest pain and the relevant ROS.*

- **O**—*Objective. The objective measures and signs we discover. Namely the vital signs and physical exam findings.*

- **A**—*Assessment of the patient's disease process. Namely, the diagnoses the patient is currently being treated for. Inclusive of the patient's current medical problems and, depending on the service, may include historical problems.*

- **P**—*Plan. The current treatment plan for the patient. The medications, labs planned, radiology studies, procedures, and discussions intended for a patient's care.*

The basics of medical chart review

Moving on to how we approach obtaining the relevant history to obtain a complete history. Sounds redundant, right? Well, it will start to make sense soon. You must review the patient's chart before seeing them to get an accurate and efficient history. Some patients have very dense charts, and navigating them will require some skill. The method of searching a chart is difficult to explain here without showing you a chart. I will do my best to describe the general principles, as one EMR will look different to another.

Once you get your first patient assigned to you, try to figure out why they are here. Usually, your senior will tell you this, or it will be documented in triage/ E.D provider notes. This is where you start. To practice this, I have an imaginary admission for you, Mr. Johnson. Quickly read the HPI, physical exam, and the management section of the E.D physician's note if available (if not available, use triage/EMS notes.)

Based on the complaint, look through his chart for relevant history. Be it through prior hospital encounters and old notes, old imaging studies, old operative notes, old procedures, external medication records, etc. Historical hospital notes are a treasure trove of history for a patient, especially H&Ps and consult notes from the relevant service. You will also need to revise the most recent lab work and imaging studies and compare them to previous studies.

Let us say Mr. Johnson is a heart failure patient; you will look at historical H&Ps, cardiology notes, echoes, stress tests, and cardiac catheterization lab reports. These will help you in managing his case now. Also, if your patient has no history at your hospital, find out where they received care prior and try to obtain records from that hospital or clinic. Prior records may wildly change a patient's management—Knowledge is King.

To briefly touch on medical bias is critical here. Just because a patient presents similarly to prior admissions does not mean it is the same disease process. Continually re-evaluate the assumptions you are making when seeing a new patient. Once you have revised the chart and your premises, you may proceed to talk to Mr. Johnson to obtain a full H&P that is relevant.

Physical examination, approach, and interpretation

Once the history taking is complete, with the help of the earlier eight points, up next is the physical exam. You must now examine the patient and obtain more information to support your preliminary diagnosis. Of course, to perform a physical exam, it goes without saying standard professional etiquette should always be maintained, obtaining consent and respecting patient dignity.

Each specialty has its specific maneuvers and techniques, but the main contribution I must add to your physical examination skills is the idea of the focused exam. I trained abroad, and our physical exam was extensive, which is helpful but time-consuming. Your goal should be to obtain the most relevant information about your patient through the exam and not miss any alarm signs.

So, Mr. Johnson needs a thorough cardiovascular exam; we can be pretty sure that he doesn't need a detailed neurological exam, right? It goes without saying you must perform a complete examination of the affected organ system, but in addition to that, you should briefly revise the other organ systems. If you are seeing a patient and do not have a solid preliminary diagnosis or differential at the very least, then I suggest you examine the patient thoroughly—like your life and their life depend on it.

It pains me to say that we do miss things. Catastrophic medical outcomes can come from missed examination signs. A blowing murmur, peritonitic abdomens, crepitus in soft tissue infections, and tense muscular compartments should come to mind. Never take the physical examination lightly because the more patients you examine, the more findings and signs you will see. The more you see, the more you will know, and the better you'll be.

Any abnormalities in labs, imaging, and physical exam should be addressed. You want to have an explanation for deviations from normal in your patient. The interpretation of all your findings is the reason for the accumulation of your experience and knowledge. This, at times, will be easy and at others, extremely difficult. We must make assumptions often; because our knowledge is imperfect. Regardless, we must exert ourselves to explain what we can, for it is in these deficiencies that we learn and improve.

Chapter 4

Babbling, Presenting Information

Once we have collected the information and started interpreting it, how do we present it? The art of presentation is a complex one. Depending on the who, what, where, when, and why you are presenting, you'll have to change *how you present*. Just as there are different modes of documentation, there are various modes of presentation.

Types of presentation, target audience, and their differences

A H&P will be a complete presentation of the patient's case from start to finish. Inclusive of all the details, as is documented in the note. This system is how you present most new patients.

A progress note will be a focused assessment of how the patient is doing today compared to yesterday.

A consultation note is like a H&P but focuses on the reason surrounding the consult and the specialty consulted. More specific and tailored for relevance.

A procedure note documents a procedure. The indications, methods, and complications, if any.

Styles of presentation and efficient communication

The first time you present to an attending should nearly always be in H&P or consultation format unless they were following the patient. If they were following, you should present it in SOAP format like a progress note. If a different attending is covering your primary attending, giving them a summary of the patient's relevant PMH, presentation, and hospitalization up to that point, then going into SOAP format is usually appreciated. They are not all-knowing beings. They need to be familiarized with patients as well.

Differences in attendings are significant. Some will prefer a H&P for each new patient they see. Overall, they will dictate how you present; what is noted above are general guidelines that seem to work for most cases. Senior residents may also have suggestions as to how you should present. Take what they say seriously. A senior resident understands how certain attendings think and how they prefer patient presentations. Take their advice as always.

The art of attention and preliminary diagnosis

General rules—do not forget about HIPPA, you should not start presenting a patient's history in public spaces. Be respectful of time; if your team is short on time, your senior may interject to summarize; do not take this personally, pay attention to how they present, and learn to become more efficient in communication. During the presentation, you are trying to reach a goal. That goal is the diagnosis—the reason for all the information gathering and discussion. So be clear when you speak and stay organized. Do not allow inconsistencies in history from the patient's end to disorient you.

You must focus on highlighting the crucial parts of the patient's history, as there will be a significant amount of information to sift through, and seniors/attendings do this intuitively. They appreciate it when you stress important points supporting your diagnosis, and this can be done using your tone, volume, and speed. Once you have presented Mr. Johnson's case to your team, they will ask: *what's your assessment and plan?*

Chapter 5

Speaking, Interpretation, and Formulation

The assessment and plan are the end of the note and the first goal of the patient encounter. It is the starting point for the patient's improvement. The first time I was asked for my assessment and plan for a patient, I just stared blankly at my senior. Here I will discuss the formulation of a complete A&P.

What is an assessment and plan? How to formulate one

I was taught to use the ABCD method in the assessment and plan, and I find it helpful in constructing a robust assessment and plan. There are different styles of organization of assessment and plans. They may be problem-based or systems-based. I prefer problem-based A&Ps; I feel they are more inclusive making us less likely to miss a diagnosis by looking at the patient as one whole with many problems that interact—instead of many different systems with different problems. Noted below is the framework for a problem-based A&P. In all honesty, once you are capable of one, you can do the other.

Assessment

- **A**—*Acute, in descending order the patient's acute problems, listed in order of severity/priority and C.C, then other acute parts of the disease process.*

- **B**—*B is for blood work; the abnormalities in the testing should be explained. If the patient's diagnoses cannot explain them, they may require further workup. May include radiological or physical examination findings.*

- **C**—*Chronic, for chronic diseases, also in descending order of active management.*

- **D**—*Diet, Disability, DVT prophylaxis, Disposition, Death.*

Structure of the assessment, reasoning, and discussion of the plan

As we can see, the critical conditions are in the beginning; this is important as other teams may skim the note only to read the assessment and plan. If they find a substantially long A&P (I am looking at the internists), they will read the beginning, assuming that is what's considered most important. The wording is critical in notation, depending on specialty, as it relates to hospital billing for both procedures and management.

You must do your best to learn the correct notation for certain diseases and procedures as you will be writing most of the notes for your service. As an example, in I.M, typing things like heart failure instead of acute on chronic systolic heart failure will get you a message from the billing department. While for surgical residents' operative notes are the true focus of note writing and CNs/PNs may be bare bones for the sake of efficiency. All notes should always address the main problems and questions one service has for another. It is a form of communication and a medicolegal document.

Next is the plan. Different physicians use different formats in the format of a note. Some people enumerate the assessment, and the respective plan follows under it. Others use signs such as the hashtag # to signify a new assessment. The first two examples are usually expected of interns. The final method is generally reserved for senior residents and beyond.

Examples of A&P structure:

i. *Acute hypoxic respiratory failure due to COPD exacerbation—*

    IV methylprednisolone 60mg q8hrs, Albuterol/ipratropium nebulized q6hrs scheduled, etc.

Or

ii. *#Acute appendicitis—*

     NPO, plan for OR, IVF rehydration, etc.

Or

iii. *Assessment:*

      1. *Acute chest pain secondary to acute NSTEMI s/p DES placement.*

      2. *Acute on chronic systolic heart failure exacerbation.*

      3. *Hypokalemia secondary to diuresis.*

Plan:

1. *Continue with aspirin, ticagrelor, metoprolol, and atorvastatin.*

2. *Pt. maintained on IV Lasix, strict intake and output, daily weights. Maintain cardiac telemetry etc.*

3. *Continue electrolyte repletion with KCL.*

I prefer to avoid enumeration as problems change in priority, thus changing the order, meaning you must also change the numbers.

My method is:

#Septic shock secondary to aspiration pneumonia—Continue IV ampicillin/sulbactam, swallow evaluation w/ speech therapy, blood and urine cultures pending, monitor fever curve, etc.

To develop the plan, you must understand how you will treat that specific condition. Here you must become adept at using the medical knowledge available to you in your mind and at your fingertips. The best method is to try and develop your own assessment and plan first, then discuss it with your senior prior to enacting it. See if they have different assessments and ask *why* they differ.

The plan is the most challenging part initially; it is the practice of medicine. It takes time, but you will start to develop your own mental algorithms of how certain diseases are treated and triage them in order of priority.

As you evolve, you'll reach a point where you are concerned about a patient's case and feel an issue hasn't been addressed. Firstly, think it through. Is there a reason why it has not been addressed? Secondly, if there isn't, evaluate the possible solutions and then direct your questions to your senior first and attending second.

When is the best time to pose your question? If it is an emergency, do not hesitate; ask immediately so as not to delay care. For non-urgent issues, it is preferable to bring up your concerns to your senior before rounds so that you can be on the same page. If they don't have a satisfactory answer, you can discuss it with your attending during rounds.

As we discussed earlier, ego is the enemy of medicine. Do not try to make yourself out to be "God's gift to medicine" and start casting doubts upon seniors and attendings based on your medical knowledge. It comes off as arrogant. You can have expansive medical knowledge and still be an amateur at patient management.

Ask for the reasoning behind clinical decision making in a respectful manner, acknowledging there is a chance you could be right and a chance you could be wrong. If you feel strongly about something, bring it up clearly. If you and the senior disagree, discuss the case with your attending. Remember, you must always stay respectful, especially in academic discussions.

Interestingly, there are two very different philosophies in the approach to a patient's ailments, and I would like to mention them here.

Hickam's dictum vs. Occam's razor

Hickam's dictum is quoted as "patients can have as many diseases as they damn well please." In more commonly used terms, each problem may have its own diagnosis. It is the counterargument to the below.

Occam's razor: "entities should not be multiplied beyond necessity," often inaccurately paraphrased as the simplest explanation is usually the best one. Applied to medicine, it means one diagnosis should explain all current medical problems.

Fusing these thought processes makes a strong clinician. Knowing when to rely on one more than the other in certain cases will come with time. They are good ideas to add to your repertoire.

All in all, your assessment and plan should be an accurate depiction of the patient's currently active medical problems, the steps being taken to correct them, and the reasoning for them occurring, if feasible. Why did your patient with diabetes go into DKA? What is the trigger? Asking why leads us to root causes, and this, in turn, leads to better treatment and outcomes for patients by preventing their recurrence.

Expectations of an intern in residency

Here we will have a brief discussion on the expectations of an intern. I discussed the roles earlier; go back to the end of Chapter 2 to revise if you have forgotten that list. Regarding all these goals and things that you must do and learn, try to take it easy. Ironic, I admit, but you need to give yourself a break. All physicians pass through a phase of feeling out of their depth. It's okay to recuperate. Take the time to appreciate that you have made it this far, and are trying to improve.

The expectations of an intern are to *try*. Not much more beyond that; it's the first and foremost expectation. Improving comes second. We all know it takes time. Team members will push you because they see your potential and want you to become independent ASAP. The faster you feel comfortable managing things alone, the closer you are to seniority. A tough beginning makes for a sweet ending, so keep at it.

The goal is that by six months, you should be quite effective. By this, I mean that you can see most patients on your list and handle their day-to-day management. I strongly suggest you aim to be completely independent for many everyday tasks by January. You may still need and should speak with your senior for advice on complex or critical cases, but you should at least have an idea of where to start the management on these scenarios by then.

I am not suggesting you run a code or do an operation on your own. I am saying: be able to see a patient, have an idea of how critical they are, what they have, how to treat, and feel comfortable with the management and documentation of bread-and-butter cases in your specialty. I think this is a reasonable goal if you apply yourself.

Yes, it may be challenging, and some people will say you have *all* your intern year to do this. I disagree; you should try to be as competent as possible as *soon* as possible. Focus on your weaknesses and work on them while you are an intern. You'll be in your senior's shoes and function as the next intern's safety net before you know it.

A brief discussion on making mistakes and dealing with them

Fear is your weapon. You should be afraid; we are all afraid. Courage is overcoming fear, not the absence of it. Senior residents and attendings are more concerned over the fearless intern than the fearful one. A fearless and ignorant person is far more dangerous to patient care than a fearful one. Use the fear of independence to spur you on. To know what patient cases scare you means you have a sense of what you don't know. Address these fears as an intern; you don't want to be overwhelmed by something you're uncomfortable with as a senior.

Dealing with fear goes hand in hand with dealing with mistakes. We all make mistakes, and no doctor practicing is perfect. We have all made the wrong call. Here lies the reason we call it the *practice of medicine*. We are forever practicing in an evolving field. You must learn from your mistakes, and beyond that, you must not permit them to paralyze you.

Reflect on them, deal with them and allow them to make you more focused. Discuss with a senior or faculty advisor about these "mistakes." Sometimes, you will be surprised to learn things about similar situations they have been through or how they would've dealt with them. *Learn,* and continue to *live.*

You are now ready to talk. Time to learn how to walk and do.

PART TWO
TO WALK AND DO

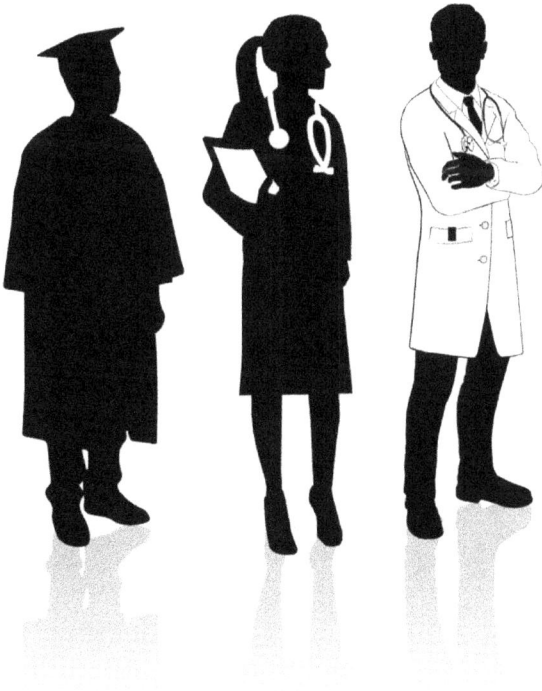

Chapter 6

Crawling, Acting with Purpose

Prioritization will become your primary concern in acting out the team's plans for patient care. What should be done first? How can you put one patient before the other? This premise may seem confusing at times, but there is a method to the madness. Allow me to list the general prioritization of patient care.

Prioritization of duties and allocation of responsibilities

1. Physically seeing patients takes precedent. If a patient is not doing well, the first thing in your mind should be seeing the patient physically. *However, you may start the management process via verbal orders until you get to the patient's bedside.* For example, a nurse calls you about your patient with new, left-sided, crushing chest pain. You should ask them to obtain an EKG and see the patient immediately. With experience, you will be able to gauge a patient and their complaint based on their active diagnoses and PMH or PSH. *Always see a patient with an alarm symptom or finding.*

2. Placing orders. To place orders is to dictate and change the treatment of a patient. Of course, seeing a patient and deciding what should be done is preferred, but this may not always be possible. Remember this; when you are told

to place an order for a patient, this should not be delayed; it *is to be done urgently*. For example, the faster you order a medication, the faster it gets sent up from the pharmacy, and the quicker the patient improves.

3. Communication with support staff. To respond to nursing staff with calls and pages will always be of utmost importance, but if you are seeing a critical patient or are in the middle of placing orders, it can wait unless it is a stat page/call then things are different. Use your sense. The best method is to answer the call/page, write down what needs to be done and evaluate if it needs to be done immediately or later. A senna order can wait; a hypotensive patient on the floor cannot.

4. Notes. Documentation is vital, as we discussed earlier, but in terms of patient care, unless it is a discharge summary or H&P, it can be done later. Always complete your documentation before leaving for the day. Try to complete them quickly as your seniors/attendings will have to place their addendums on your note, and the earlier it is done, the better. DC summaries can be started from the day of admission to expedite discharge when the patient is ready. Some programs will require writing both a PN and DC summary on discharge day.

5. Housework. Before leaving for the day, always ensure you have updated the handoff, signed out to the appropriate people, and tied up any loose ends possible. Order morning labs, revise orders and see if new notes are available with new recommendations for patient management. Discuss with your senior before enacting those new recommendations. Despite your shift ending, your peers will judge you if you walk out on a crashing patient mid-management. If you speak to the oncoming team and plan on transferring care to them, then you may go. Always do your best to help

each other out. You will be in their position at some point in residency.

This framework can be applied to most services and shifts: coming in, seeing your patients, managing them, continuing care, and ensuring their care moves forward tomorrow. If you remember our prior discussion, you are part of a team. You do not carry the "list" on your own. You should be able to allocate responsibility to others to help you manage. For you, these are your medical students.

You can give your medical students tasks to complete so that they can also learn and progress to be successful interns. Medical students can make phone calls, assist with procedures, speak with CMs and SWs, place orders with your supervision, and write billable notes (MS-4, not MS-3s). They can genuinely offload some of your responsibilities, and this will serve to give them a realistic experience of the rotation. Try to be fair; they have their limits and still have class requirements, etc. Do not overload the medical students to avoid work (or empower your ego); this will come back to bite you.

The art of time management, rhythm, and flow

Managing your time while doing all these things will prove difficult. Multitasking is the friend of an intern. Walking, talking, and placing orders while performing other tasks are instrumental skills. Practice makes perfect, and once you become more familiar with the EMR you will become more efficient. As always, be respectful and tactful of when and where you are doing something. Patients do not appreciate distracted doctors during their encounters.

You will need to develop a routine for each rotation you work on. My practice is getting sign-out in the morning, revising my team's patients' available vitals, lab work, and notes quickly, and then doing what we call pre-rounds. Seeing your patients early is vital, as the earlier they are seen, the earlier things can be addressed. If your residency has a morning report, try to see your patients before the start of the morning report, if allowed.

Always see patients in priority of severity first and foremost; it is a golden rule: *the sickest are seen first.* If you have a patient who had a CRT overnight resulting in significantly changed management, see them first. As the primary team, you know the patient better and understand their case better than the covering team. Not all CRTs are genuinely critical, and so you must learn how to gauge the unwell vs. the well. For example, a patient who vomited blood is someone you must see first; they have priority over the patient discharging home today.

Overall, the prioritization of patient care, as you can see, has to do with how ill the patient is, but that is not the *only* scenario. You must also focus on helping the hospital machinery work efficiently, namely, discharging patients early. This serves to support all patients, not just our own. Hospital beds are a precious commodity, and the faster we can get people who need them in them, the better.

This prioritization of patients will lead to the rhythm and flow of your workday. You will get a sense of what needs to be done first, second and third. The importance of establishing this rhythm or routine is good for you too. You need to be able to eat, drink and just be human; this is just as important as caring for patients.

It is harder to care for others if *you* are not well. Prioritize yourself when you can, as we are humans, not machines. Commonly residents will eat lunch during their conferences and refuel with snacks, coffee, etc., during their workday. Be efficient with your use of time. Get your rhythm, feel your flow, and continue moving forward.

Chapter 7

Cruising, Seeing Patients

Once you have a framework for seeing patients, you should be asking yourself, what about if I receive multiple patients at once? How are patients assigned anyway? Who decided all this? Here we will briefly touch on general assignment methods and patient priority.

Assignment methods, priority, triaging by severity

The best way to understand this is from a patient's point of view. Thus, let us change our viewpoint for this chapter; you are now a patient. You are evaluated in triage, and based on their criteria for severity, you will be assigned to a particular E.D unit. In the E.D unit, an attending and possibly residents/PAs will be working as the providers there. The E.D nurses will take an initial set of vitals, and with triage's preliminary history from you, the providers are ready to see you. They begin their workup, see you, and start stabilizing and initially managing your case.

If they deem your case severe enough that you need admission, they will call the respective service and discuss your case to admit you. Based on your disease process or needs, you'll be sent to a respective hospital floor. You will also be assigned a priority of evaluation based on severity. Systems differ, but something like

Priority 1 (P1), P2, and P3 will serve to alert the team that you must be evaluated within a specific timeframe.

A senior resident or a staff member from the admitting office will then assign the resident to see you. Once you are in your bed, the nursing staff from that floor will call or page the assigned resident or intern for your orders. They will come, see you and take your H&P. The order may differ; some senior residents prefer to see patients before the intern. Some residents will see you in the E.D and some will wait until " you hit the floor." You will have answered two sets of similar questions and can now rest. The residents will place your management plan orders and discuss your care with an attending. This is generally the system for the admitting service.

For consult services, though, patients appear on a list and should be seen based on the priority or timing of the consult. A stat/urgent consult may be an emergency and usually requires physician-to-physician communication about the case. A routine consult means the patient should be seen within 24 hours of the order's placement. Depending on the service, an intern can see a consult, with or without a senior. The case will be discussed with the attending, and they will make final management decisions or recommendations. As discussed earlier, we should prioritize a patient with a pending discharge consult over a routine consult. Timeliness all falls on the primary team ordering consults correctly. Necrotizing fasciitis is a STAT consult for the general surgery team; it is not to be placed routine.

Cross-coverage, alarm symptoms and signs, tips, and tricks

Now that you understand the assignment system, just apply the rules mentioned earlier in terms of seeing these patients—sickest sooner and well can wait. Triaging and managing multiple critical patients can be difficult. If you are ever in this situation, ask for help from your senior or teammates. Do not try to handle everything on your own. You can't physically be at three bedsides at once. For this reason, we work as a team in inpatient care.

Regarding being a team, remember a residency program is akin to a machine. Many moving parts are functioning while others rest and vice versa. How do we care for patients that are not our own? This question brings us to the discussion of cross-coverage. You will likely hold the service pager when you or your team are on call. Cross-coverage means covering calls and pages for the patients admitted to the service and the multiple teams working under it. This role is not an easy one, and although your focus is being there for emergencies, you must act and address new problems all the time. Patient care does not follow a schedule of 9–5; it is 24/7.

When carrying the cross-coverage pager, you may have other roles, such as admitting new patients. Always try to manage both simultaneously while still prioritizing. You may be asked by nurses about pretty much anything. If it is non-urgent, it is okay to tell them; that you will call back if you are busy. Things like ordering a diet, IVF, extra insulin on top of ISS for hyperglycemia, or holding medications for one reason or another will all be routed to you. You will have to make decisions quickly for these common problems.

Do not worry; you will grow accustomed to this with time, and run-of-the-mill calls can be managed without much deliberation. For example, you do not need to look up a patient's LFTS to give them acetaminophen if they are admitted for pneumonia. Be careful, though, with sedating and medicating patients for specific problems. Things like agitation, and pain beyond the basic OTC meds, may be disease-specific. In these cases, it is vital to look at the hand-off briefly and ask for a patient's creatinine to ensure that the patient can receive certain medications. A patient with acute kidney injury should not be given NSAIDs, if possible, and so on.

Call your senior if you run into an issue that you don't know how to handle or a complex case. Their experience can also help navigate difficult patients or even nursing staff situations if need be. Your role is to treat patients; you are not responsible for bed assignments and the like.

A brief word on alarm symptoms. A patient's disease process rarely picks a convenient time or place. They may choose to decompensate at any time in any manner. We should be ready to manage these situations to the best of our abilities. Should you get called/paged about an alarm symptom or sign, see that patient, and contact your senior once you've started preliminary testing and management.

Scenarios like severe chest or abdominal pain, bloody vomiting/bowel movements, new-onset neurological deficits, and severely abnormal vital signs must be addressed quickly. These are often the criteria for a CRT as well. Successful management of these problems might save that patient from an ICU transfer or cardiorespiratory arrest.

Remember, nursing staff are our eyes and ears; they spend more time at the bedside than we do and are more familiar with the patient than we are at times. If they are concerned, you should be concerned, allowing for differences in personalities and training, etc. Do not shrug off a concerned nurse or even a patient's family member. Try to address everyone's concerns if possible. At the end of the day, physicians will always have the "Captain of the ship" responsibility. That makes us not only responsible for the care of the patient but also for the people who care for and advocate for that patient.

Some tips and tricks are useful in this regard. As a daytime physician, try to communicate the patient's condition and care plan to the family and nursing staff. These discussions will help offload the night team from such matters. Also, as I said earlier, use verbal orders to your advantage. Nurses will ask for the order, verbal read-back, and your name. They can get started giving the patient medications and ordering simple tests while you review the chart and come to see the patient.

Chapter 8
Walking, Placing Orders

Placing orders. I have discussed the importance of this time and time again. Now to explain how it is done. EMRs do not vary much on how to place orders as much as they do on the name of orders. For example: Duplex vs. doppler vs. U/S of the lower extremity.

How to place an order, priority, route, and timing

The general method is going to the area of the chart called orders. Clicking on either the new order button or a + sign. Once you have chosen your order, you must then choose the who, what, why, where and when of the order. Allow me to demonstrate with three examples of different order types.

Ordering a medication:

1. *Type in the medication's pharmaceutical or trade name into the search bar. Select the medication, right-click to modify, or double-click the order itself. What is being given?*

2. *Choose the priority: STAT, routine, timed, etc. How soon should this be given?*

3. *Then the route: PO, IV, via feeding tube, rectally. How should this be given?*

4. *Then the time or schedule. When should this be given?*

5. *Doses: in mg/g/ml etc. How much of this is to be given?*

6. *Duration: in doses, days, occurrences, or once. How long will this be given for?*

After filling all this out, you must click the sign button to finalize the order. You may see a pop-up for allergies and interactions; read through these quickly. They may or may not be clinically relevant. Some EMRs require you to click refresh for the order to be fully activated in the patient's chart.

Ordering an imaging study:

1. *Enter the type of study or name in the search bar. Select it, right-click to modify, or double-click the order itself. What is being done?*

2. *Choose the indication-populated list of choices or buttons, and leave a brief explanation in the comment section if other. Why is this being done?*

3. *Priority: STAT, routine, pending DC, timed, AM, etc. How soon should this be done?*

4. *Choose the type: laterality, focus, region, etc. Where should this be done? Additionally, you must choose with or without contrast: oral or IV?*

5. *Questions on obstructive hardware will vary by study. Example: MRIs and old pacemakers. Reactions to contrast are also a concern; if not severe, pre-medicate the pt.*

Ordering a procedure:

1. *Enter the procedure's name or type in the search bar. Select it, right-click modify or double-click the order itself. What is being done?*

2. *Choose the indication. From a populated list of choices or buttons, leave a brief explanation in the comment section if "Other" is chosen. Why is this being done?*

3. *Priority: STAT, routine, pending DC, timed, AM, etc. How soon should this be done?*

4. *Then choose the type: laterality, focus, region, etc. Where should this be done? Also, prohibitive points for the procedure, on therapeutic anticoagulation (not DVT ppx), a patient can't give consent, etc., may be mentioned in comments or there could be options.*

Types of orders and order sets

This construct for placing an order applies to other types of orders, such as lab tests, consults, nursing orders, and communication orders. There are also miscellaneous orders for specific tests that are rarely ordered. Overall, these assist in specifying particular treatment goals, bedside procedures, or management techniques for a patient.

Now to touch on an essential point regarding STAT orders. The sequence of events in the background is rapid, depending on the order. Suppose you order a STAT CT. The imaging department will call the nurse for the transport of the patient and try to clear the table for the scan. Imagine being at the end of that call and not knowing your pt. is going for a STAT CT Abd/Pelvis w/contrast for bowel perforation.

You must communicate with nursing staff if something emergent needs to be done with your pt. and something needs to be done STAT. It will streamline care and allow the orders placed to occur quickly. Trust me; if it says STAT and you do not communicate to other team members, more often than not, there will be delays.

A brief word on procedures. Performing procedures is the hallmark of some residencies and a rarity for others. The best practice for learning how to do a procedure is first to understand it in theory. Learning the indications, contraindications and complications comes first, then the tools and methodology of the procedure, in and of itself, come second.

Depending on your specialty, you may never perform a procedure, it will be expected of you daily, or it is an occasional occurrence. What is important is the method with which you approach learning a procedure. You should be enthusiastic, but do not be over-confident in your capabilities. Take things slowly. The old adage of "watch one, do one, teach one" is useful in this regard. Learn first, practice second. Developing procedural competence takes practice and an open mind. So, learn from your seniors and assist when you can.

My suggestion is to use the resources available to you. Your seniors, online videos, the simulation lab, and even the procedural kit in and of itself are all banks of knowledge. This applies to bedside procedures, such as central lines, arterial lines, peripheral IV placements, thoracentesis, paracentesis, etc.

For non-surgical residencies, ultrasound competence is becoming more and more relevant for procedures. Learning to use a bedside U/S is a skill that is growing in popularity, so study it when you can. Regarding surgical residencies, in addition to U/S skills, proficiency in suturing and laparoscopic techniques are vital, but nothing supersedes O.R training. Dedication and diligence make for a solid proceduralist.

Turning back to the EMR now, the general organization of an order section of the chart will be along the lines of medications—active and prn, diet, code status, consults, nursing orders, imaging studies, lab studies, and planned procedures or special tests. Always double-check after placing an order that it went through correctly and is active. To see if a medication has been given before or not, look at the MAR, usually found in another part of the chart.

Order sets are tools provided through the joint work of hospital management and the EMR to standardize orders for specific diseases or procedures. They are a long list of orders, organized with different options to facilitate management. There will be general admission order sets and specific order sets for procedures or admissions, like a heart failure order set. Go through the order sets and think about why certain orders are in one set, but not the other. For example, a lactate level is in a sepsis order set but not in a stroke order set. Order sets are valuable sources of information for guideline-directed management and hospital protocol.

Once you have selected all the relevant orders from the order set, sign the order set and revise the active orders for your patient. Depending on EMR, the standalone orders and order set choices may be signed and held to be released at a future point in time, or you must refresh the chart to activate the orders.

Care team communications

Orders are not only for the indications noted above, but also include consults to facilitate team communication in the hospital for a patient's case. Let us say you have ordered a consult, and that team has seen your patient, but you still have questions for them. How do you reach them?

There is a myriad of apps for HIPPA compliant messaging; using these will be helpful if your hospital provides them. Simply type in your message to the consultant or someone on their team and wait for a response. Always be respectful. If possible, as a resident, speak to the resident or fellow on service instead of going to the attending immediately.

If your attending asks you to communicate to the attending, then do so; it is also acceptable to speak to them directly if they are managing that service alone. These suggestions are just common courtesy. Also, always aim to talk to the person who saw your patient as some consulting services have multiple teams.

If your hospital doesn't employ a messaging application, you can still contact the physician the old-fashioned way, be it by pager, hospital phone, or even HIPPA compliant email. Some EMRs do have messaging applications within them from provider to provider. When speaking with other teams and physicians, try to learn from them as well—don't be afraid to ask for the reasoning behind a decision.

Chapter 9

Running, Writing Notes

We have touched on the types of notes prior and the framework for writing them. Here we will discuss being efficient in note writing. This is where most interns spend time. Let's quickly revise the types of notes, namely: PNs, H&Ps, CNs, DC summaries, and operative/ procedure notes. You must first choose the correct note type, and then we can move on to writing the note.

Types of notes, significance, and etiquette

We have spoken about the types of notes, but each of these notes has its nuances and requirements. The most common notes are straightforward in this regard, and learning billing requirements are helpful but beyond the scope of this book. Overall using the eight points for a H&P or consult note and having enough ROS/ PE on a PN (SOAP) note will suffice.

Now, for specific notes like a procedure note, there is a standard note type to be selected, and the documentation of any note is linked to billing, so doing this correctly is important. Standard protocol dictates that you include the indication of the procedure, if consent was obtained or waived, and the type of procedure in the note.

There is another note that we must mention here: the death note. A death note, or expiration note, is documentation of the patient's death exam and family discussion. It must include the death exam, which will vary but generally mentions absent breath sounds, heart sounds, etc. It should also include whether the family or next of kin wishes to have an autopsy performed. Hospital policy regarding autopsies varies but always speak with nursing/ medical examiner if an autopsy is obligatory in your patient's case. A patient who passes during an admission needs both an expiration note and a DC summary note completed.

Remember when we mentioned revising old notes for chart review? This technique can be an immense resource for writing your new note, but there is an etiquette to using old information for a new encounter. That being said, you should always confirm what was historically documented if possible.

You should not copy and paste somebody's documentation into your notation without attributing it to them or asking their permission. I do not suggest copying old notes from other physicians except for particular scenarios. You must use your judgment, but as an intern, you should always try to write your own notes as this is how you get better at it.

When writing your note, remember to respect the patient, the hospital staff, and even co-patients. Patients can read notes; this should not make you afraid but should make you conscious of the wording you use. Also, notes need to be used as medicolegal documents at times, and your note may be used in a court case at some point. As we can see the significance of a note lies in the documentation of the patient's care and can even be a future reference for their hospital admissions.

Ensure your documentation is an accurate and honest account of the patient's condition and discussions. We practice at a difficult time; trust in physicians and science is dangerously low. Ensuring you are transparent with patients in communication and documentation will save you from trouble in your career. A sloppy note that is copy/pasted, outdated and irrelevant can easily lead anybody to blame a physician for a bad outcome.

How to be efficient, the art of copy & paste

Certain parts of a note do not vary much depending on the patient's case. You should always ask the appropriate questions, but you do not need to retype everything again. The PMH/PSH/FH/allergies and physical exam need only be revised and then updated if confirmed. For example: a patient with an AKA of their left leg will not have a new leg with our current medical capabilities.

Also, for a patient you see and write progress notes daily about, it is okay to copy and paste your note. *You must update it, as it should reflect the care and changes noted that day.* To do this efficiently, you should cut out the excess. I am against noting the trend of lab results in your note. That is present in the lab region of the chart; why redouble that? Instead, describe trends, for example: down-trending, up-trending, resolved, worsening, etc.

Shortcuts, addendums, and differences

At times there are additional tools to help speed up the note-writing process. These notation shortcuts include templates or phrases (can be a word or any keyboard symbol.) These link to prior saved templates for a whole note, specific parts of a note, or procedures. There are also dictation applications that convert speech to text using deep learning artificial intelligence. Not all EMRs and hospitals provide these applications and services.

For example, here is an imaginary "star" phrase, typing: *OAROS would automatically fill that space on the note where the cursor lies with my review of systems.

- **Constitutional:** *No Fever, No Chills, No Sweats, No Weight Loss, No Change in Appetite*

- **Neurological:** *No Headache, No Dizziness, No Syncope, No Numbness, No Tingling*

- **Cardiovascular:** *No Chest Pain, No Palpitations, No Leg Swelling*

- **Respiratory:** *No Shortness of Breath, No Cough*

- **Abdomen:** *No Abdominal Pain, No Nausea, No Vomiting, No Diarrhea, No Constipation*

- **Genitourinary:** *No Dysuria, No Hematuria, No Incontinence*

- **Musculoskeletal:** *No Joint Pain, No Joint Swelling, No Skin Rash*

- **Psychiatric:** *No Changes in Mood, No Hallucinations*

These must, of course, be updated and corrected to reflect the patient's case accurately. They save time, and I strongly suggest using these phrases. Make as many personalized ones as you wish to benefit from. There are also templates through which you can click on choices for your review of systems: choosing yes and no, entering details, etc. I have found them more cumbersome than helpful, except for documenting procedures.

Once your notes are completed, you must have them co-signed by an attending. Depending on your residency, your senior may need to add what is called an addendum to your note. These can be extensive or short, like "agree with intern A&P." Different specialties will also have different practices. Some programs choose to forward notes for signature to attendings and for review to seniors. Always sign your notes at the end after your attending addends them.

If dictation is available at your hospital, *use dictation even if you are unfamiliar with it.* It will save you time, and the more you use it, the better it gets at understanding you. You can always type out your notes, but dictation is faster, although it may be inaccurate and have more typos. If you learn to use the voice commands as well, the time saved dictating will be exponentially more than the time wasted proofreading.

Chapter 10

Sitting, Continuous Care.

Sit down; you can almost relax since you have learned to think, talk, and walk like a resident. You have done what has been asked of you. Before you can fully kick back, you should revise your patients for the day and ensure things are taken care of for tomorrow.

Even if you are not working the next day, or a different team will be picking up the patient, certain things must be taken care of. These are the housework or list management footnotes for brief revision.

Patient revision, future testing, and planning

These include lab orders for the morning labs. These are meant to continue monitoring current lab abnormalities that are being watched or treated. You should always try to do what's best for the patient, and at times, that is nothing. If a patient is pending placement in the hospital after completing treatment, pending a SAR bed, and doing well, then why get daily blood work? It is both painful and costly for the patient. Do not order tests just for the sake of ordering them. Have a *reason* for what you do.

Hand-off and sign-out should also be done well. Sign-out, as we mentioned, is a summary of the patient's hospitalization up to that point and is used for transfer of patients or cross coverage. The hand-off is the document that contains the sign-out of a patient. The sign-out should include important information about the patient—not every detail of their life and hospitalization.

It is a need-to-know form of summary. Being excessive in sign-out will waste both your time and the covering resident's time. Be focused and pertinent on what needs to be conveyed for that specific patient. In general, it should be similar in the beginning to an HPI.

Start with the name, age, and pertinent PMH or PSH, C.C, hospitalization summary, treatment course, code status, and clinical status. Regarding clinical status, it is a crucial aspect of sign-out. What is meant by clinical status is: are they stable or unstable? All in all, should they be concerned about this patient? You need to communicate this exceptionally well if that is the case.

Furthermore, let the covering team know if you expect blood work or test results that need to be followed. Any critical lab results or imaging results will be relayed to the covering team. As an intern covering, if you receive a critical result, inform your senior. This is an issue that must be taken care of promptly. For example, a lactic acid level of 9 mmol/L or potassium of 7 mmol/L are abnormalities that need to be addressed immediately as they may warrant drastic changes in management, like ICU transfer or dialysis.

Having precautionary measures in place so that the covering team does not waste precious time is always appreciated. For example, you have a patient with postoperative bleeding. The patient's hemoglobin is 7.3 gm/dl on their last CBC. If they are still bleeding, you anticipate they'll need a blood transfusion. Then you should order a type and screen, order blood products on hold, and obtain transfusion consent so that when the next H&H shows a Hb of 6.1 gm/dl, they can order the unit of blood and move on.

Important discussions and moving forward

It goes without saying that important discussions with patients/ their health care proxy (HCP) or family members should be documented. It helps everyone to understand the plan and goal of patient care. If the patient is not doing well and opts for hospice or comfort care, this should be discussed with their family/HCP and be documented accordingly.

I have brought up code status a few times, and it is finally time to address it. It was defined as the course of action if a patient has cardio-respiratory arrest. Any discussion held with a patient or HCP regarding a change in code status should be documented well in the chart. The patient must be competent and have the capacity to make such a decision. If they do not, it falls on the HCP.

Code status should be addressed on admission. There will always be a physical form that needs to be filled out if the patient or HCP opts for DNR/DNI. Do your best to understand people's choices but also be aware of your surroundings. People can get very emotional if this discussion is not handled correctly.

For patients who leave the hospital AMA, you should try to counsel them on staying if possible. Not all patients can leave AMA. Suicidal ideation or intoxicated patients, for example, are forced to remain admitted ("Committed") until they have decision-making capacity.

At the end of your workday is the finish line. You have seen your patients, enacted plans, and prepared your patients for continuous care. This is the goal of your intern year—to be able to complete these tasks with ease while learning the practical medicine behind the management.

The transition to seniority is quite abrupt—one day, you *are* an intern, and the next, you *have* an intern. If you combine these skills and techniques with the ongoing acquisition of medical knowledge, I can assure you your transition to seniority will be smooth. Residency is high-pace and, at times, high stress, but nowhere else in the world have I seen such competent physicians developed in such a short span of time.

Every journey has an end, and this is the end of your intern workday. Do this a couple hundred more times, and you'll stand at the end of your intern year. If you can abide by the doctrines I have set forth, I have no doubt you will succeed during residency. Please continue to practice and believe in the nobility of our profession. Although the road does get dark at times, look for light on your way. Be it a goal, a memory, a patient, or a situation. Even mushroom clouds have silver linings.

Chapter 11

Finish Line. Evolution.

Once you have reached the goal of becoming an efficient, accurate, and safe intern, you can progress to becoming a stellar resident. The best methodology is to continue the same work ethic from your intern year throughout your progression in residency. Humility goes a long way, and teaching others will always add to your wealth of knowledge. The more you practice, the more you can give to both patients and junior physicians.

Final thoughts

Let's now touch upon the evaluations you obtain during your rotations. In the USA, there is a 360-degree modality of evaluation. Everyone on the team evaluates each other, from the medical student, the intern, and the senior resident to the attending. As an intern, one of the most valuable resources for improving will be constructive criticism in your evaluations.

To better yourself, why wait on the evaluation? During your rotations, you can privately ask how you are doing to the team members. They can give you pointers on what to work on before your evaluation. If you can make improvements before your evaluation, it will be that much better.

The program leadership revises your evaluations, and you are judged based on your postgraduate year and other metrics set by the ACGME. The stronger the evaluation, the stronger the resident you seem to be. Based on your evaluations, you may be offered more responsibilities in the residency as you progress, such as Chief Resident. These will also help build up your skills and reputation for your immediate and future goals.

The Future

No matter what path you may take, being a solid resident will always be helpful in your career. Roles such as Chief Resident, in resident governance, etc., will look strong on your C.V and help propel you to new heights. Fellowship applications you make in the future will prompt people to look deeply at how you did in residency. The better you did, the better they can expect you to do with them.

Aspirations and goals are difficult to discern in residency; some people have no idea, while others have their hearts set on a sub-subspecialty. People differ and have varying comfort levels with committing to a specific specialty early in training. This is normal. Do not compound stress on yourself because you do not *precisely* know what you want to be upon graduation. You have time to explore.

This is not to say that having a specific goal is necessarily a bad thing. On the contrary, knowing what you want to do for fellowship or for a career after residency can help you excel and focus on specific topics. Overall, once you have a long-term goal, you can make short-term targets.

Regarding fellowship, distinguishing yourself as a resident is imperative. Connecting with consultants and fellows during residency will also be an immense resource. Displaying your interest with research and outside rotations will add more and more weight to your application and, as such, is strongly suggested for a competitive fellowship.

In addition to that, working with your co-residents on research projects and abstract presentations are enjoyable and invaluable experiences, especially if you present at a conference. If you decide to take another route, be it academic or private practice, do not hesitate to discuss with your mentors for advice and guidance on how to succeed. They can give pointers on billing, how to operate a clinic efficiently, etc.

Enough about expectations and goals and rules; I hope you have enjoyed reading this book as much as I have enjoyed writing it. It brought pleasant and funny stories to mind from my residency. It is an arduous journey but well worth the struggle. I am forever indebted to my seniors, attendings, and patients for the medical knowledge and values instilled in me. I hope that this guide has given you a piece of that.

I urge you to make the most of your time in training. Learn and teach as much as you can, stay humble, and keep at it. The field of medicine may be demanding, but it is equally rewarding. To quote Sir Isaac Newton—"If I have seen further, it is by standing on the shoulders of giants." We must strive to become steppingstones to further the view into the ever-expanding horizon of medical knowledge.

So go on—walk, talk, and do. Start your medical career journey well prepared and enjoy the trip.

Index

T

V

W

X

www.ingramcontent.com/pod-product-compliance
Lightning Source LLC
Chambersburg PA
CBHW071457210326
41597CB00018B/2581